Isometric Exercises for Pain Relief

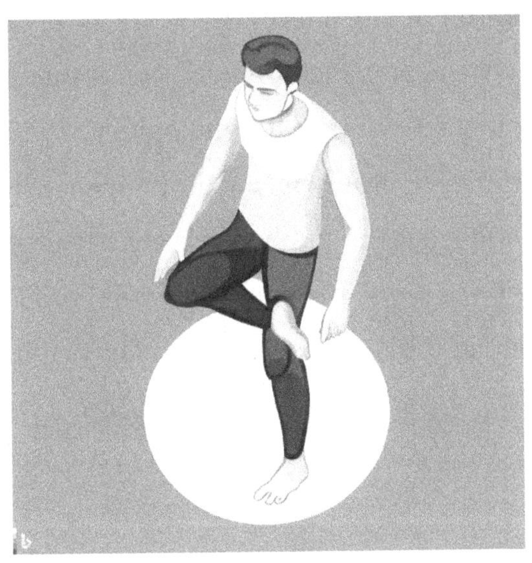

How to Build Strength and Endurance Without Moving

Patrick Moore

Table of Contents

Introduction

Welcome to "Isometric Exercises for Pain Relief: How to Build Strength and Endurance Without Moving." This book is designed to introduce you to the world of isometric exercises and their incredible potential for relieving pain while simultaneously improving your strength and endurance. Isometric exercises involve contracting your muscles without joint movement, making them ideal for individuals with chronic pain, injuries, or limited mobility.

In this comprehensive guide, we will explore the numerous benefits of isometric exercises, including their ability to reduce pain, increase muscle tone, and enhance overall physical performance. You will discover a wide range of targeted exercises for different areas of the body, along with step-by-step instructions on proper form and technique. Furthermore, we will delve into advanced techniques, program design, and practical tips for maximising results.

Whether you are seeking relief from pain or aiming to improve your physical fitness, this book will provide you with the knowledge and tools necessary to incorporate isometric exercises into your daily life effectively.

Understanding Isometric Exercises

In order to fully benefit from isometric exercises, it is essential to have a solid understanding of their principles and how they differ from other forms of physical activity. Isometric exercises involve the contraction of specific muscles without any accompanying joint movement. Unlike dynamic exercises that involve repetitive motions, isometric exercises require you to hold a static position while exerting force against an immovable object or resisting against your own body weight.

The key concept behind isometric exercises lies in the muscle contraction and the resulting tension generated within the targeted muscles. When you perform an isometric exercise, the muscle fibers engage and exert force, but there is no visible movement at the joint. This static contraction places a significant load on the muscle, activating a high number of motor units and recruiting a larger portion of muscle fibers compared to other types of exercises.

During an isometric exercise, your muscle fibers generate tension and experience an increase in intra-muscular pressure. This elevated pressure enhances blood flow to the targeted muscle, delivering oxygen and essential nutrients. Additionally, isometric exercises activate the central nervous system, leading to an increase in neural drive and improved motor unit recruitment. This neurological adaptation contributes to the development of strength and power in the engaged muscles.

By understanding the fundamental principles of isometric exercises, you can effectively harness their benefits for strength development, muscle toning, and injury prevention. Throughout this book, we will delve deeper into the specific techniques, exercises, and programs that will empower you to incorporate isometric exercises into your routine and experience the positive impact they can have on your overall fitness and well-being.

Benefits of Isometric Exercises for Pain Relief

Isometric exercises offer a range of significant benefits for individuals seeking relief from pain. By incorporating these exercises into your routine, you can effectively manage and reduce pain while improving your overall physical well-being. Here are some key advantages of isometric exercises for pain relief:

1. *Targeted Muscle Strengthening:* Isometric exercises allow you to focus on specific muscle groups without putting excessive strain on your joints. By strengthening these muscles, you can provide better support and stability to the surrounding joints, reducing pain caused by weakness or imbalances.

2. *Enhanced Muscle Endurance:* Isometric exercises improve muscle endurance by increasing the time your muscles can sustain a contraction. This increased endurance is particularly beneficial for individuals with chronic pain, as it helps them perform daily activities with less discomfort and fatigue.

3. *Joint Stability and Protection:* Isometric exercises promote joint stability by strengthening the muscles and connective tissues surrounding the joints. This added stability can alleviate pain caused by joint instability, such as in conditions like osteoarthritis or ligament injuries.

4. *Improved Posture and Alignment:* Isometric exercises engage the core muscles, promoting better posture and alignment. By strengthening the core muscles, you can alleviate pain in the neck, back, and shoulders, which is often associated with poor posture.

5. *Reduced Muscle Tension:* Isometric exercises help release tension and relax muscles. By engaging in these exercises, you can relieve muscular tightness and spasms, which are common sources of pain and discomfort.

6. *Low-Impact Option:* Isometric exercises are low-impact, making them suitable for individuals with joint pain or injuries. They provide an opportunity to strengthen and condition muscles without placing excessive stress on the joints.

How Isometric Exercises Can Help Build Strength and Endurance

Isometric exercises are not only effective for pain relief, but they also offer significant benefits in building strength and endurance. Incorporating these exercises into your fitness routine can help you develop muscular strength, increase endurance, and improve overall physical performance. Here's how isometric exercises contribute to building strength and endurance:

1. *Muscle Fiber Recruitment:* Isometric exercises activate a large number of muscle fibers simultaneously. By holding a static position and exerting force against resistance, you engage a significant portion of your muscle fibers, leading to increased muscle activation and recruitment. This recruitment stimulates muscle growth and strength development.

2. *Overcoming Plateaus:* Isometric exercises can help break through strength plateaus that may occur with traditional dynamic exercises. By introducing isometric holds, you challenge your muscles in a different way, promoting further strength gains. This variation can be especially beneficial for individuals who have reached a plateau in their strength training journey.

3. Time Under Tension: Isometric exercises require you to hold a contraction for a specific duration, leading to an extended time under tension for the muscles. This prolonged contraction stimulates muscle fibers, promoting their growth and enhancing muscular endurance.

4. Full Body Engagement: Many isometric exercises engage multiple muscle groups simultaneously, providing a full-body workout. These exercises require stabilisation and activation of various muscles, leading to overall strength development and improved functional fitness.

5. Increased Joint Stability: Isometric exercises strengthen the muscles around the joints, providing enhanced stability and support. This increased stability can help protect the joints during dynamic movements, allowing you to perform exercises with better form and reduced risk of injury.

6. Progressive Overload: Isometric exercises can be easily adjusted to increase the level of difficulty and challenge. By gradually increasing the intensity or duration of the holds, you can progressively overload your muscles, stimulating further strength and endurance gains.

Incorporating isometric exercises into your training regimen can complement traditional strength and endurance exercises, providing a well-rounded approach to fitness. It is important to consult with a fitness professional to ensure proper form and technique, as well as to design a tailored program that aligns with your specific goals and fitness level.

Chapter 2

Getting Started with Isometric Exercises

Safety Precautions and Considerations

Before diving into isometric exercises, it's crucial to understand the safety precautions and considerations associated with this form of physical activity. By following these guidelines, you can ensure a safe and effective workout experience. Here are some key safety precautions and considerations to keep in mind:

1. Consult with a Healthcare Professional: If you have any pre-existing medical conditions or concerns, it's important to consult with a healthcare professional before starting any exercise program, including isometric exercises. They can provide personalized advice and recommendations based on your specific needs and medical history.

2. *Warm-up and Cool-down:* Prior to engaging in isometric exercises, it's essential to warm up your muscles and prepare your body for the workout. Perform dynamic stretches or light aerobic activities to increase blood flow and loosen up the muscles. Similarly, remember to cool down and stretch after your workout to promote muscle recovery and prevent post-exercise soreness.

3. *Proper Form and Technique:* Pay careful attention to your form and technique during isometric exercises. Proper alignment and positioning are crucial to target the intended muscles and avoid unnecessary strain or injury. Consider seeking guidance from a qualified trainer or fitness professional to ensure you are performing the exercises correctly.

4. *Gradual Progression:* Start with exercises that match your current fitness level and gradually progress to more challenging variations. Avoid pushing yourself too hard or attempting exercises that are beyond your capabilities, as it may lead to injury. Progression should be gradual and based on your individual strength and comfort level.

5. *Listen to Your Body:* Pay attention to your body's signals during the workout. If you experience sharp pain, dizziness, or unusual discomfort, stop the exercise immediately. It's essential to differentiate between the normal feeling of muscle fatigue and pain that indicates potential injury. If in doubt, consult with a healthcare professional.

6. Breathing and Hydration: Maintain proper breathing techniques throughout the exercises. Exhale during the contraction phase and inhale during the relaxation phase. Additionally, stay hydrated by drinking an adequate amount of water before, during, and after your workout.

7. Rest and Recovery: Allow your body ample time to rest and recover between exercise sessions. Overtraining can lead to fatigue, decreased performance, and an increased risk of injury. Incorporate rest days into your routine to promote muscle recovery and optimize your overall fitness progress.

By following these safety precautions and considerations, you can minimise the risk of injury and ensure a safe and effective start to your journey with isometric exercises. Remember, safety should always be a top priority when engaging in any form of physical activity.

Equipment Needed for Isometric Exercises

One of the great advantages of isometric exercises is that they can be performed with minimal equipment, making them accessible for people of all fitness levels and budgets. While many isometric exercises require no equipment at all, there are a few optional pieces of equipment that can enhance your workout experience. Here are some common equipment options for isometric exercises:

1. Exercise Mat: An exercise mat provides a comfortable and supportive surface for performing floor-based isometric exercises, such as planks or bridge exercises. It helps cushion your body and provides grip, ensuring stability during the holds.

2. Resistance Bands: Resistance bands are versatile and affordable tools that can add an extra challenge to your isometric exercises. They provide external resistance, increasing the intensity of the muscle contractions. Resistance bands can be used for various exercises, including bicep curls, squats, or shoulder exercises.

3. Stability Ball: Also known as an exercise or Swiss ball, a stability ball can be used to add instability to your isometric exercises. By incorporating a stability ball, you engage more muscles to maintain balance and stability during the holds. It can be used for exercises like wall sits, planks, or core strengthening exercises.

4. Hand Grippers: Hand grippers are small, handheld devices designed to strengthen the muscles in your hands and forearms. They can be particularly useful for individuals looking to improve grip strength or for rehabilitation purposes.

5. Yoga Blocks: Yoga blocks can be utilised to modify the difficulty of certain isometric exercises. By adjusting the height or position of the blocks, you can tailor the exercise to your current fitness level and gradually progress as you get stronger.

It's important to note that while these equipment options can enhance your isometric workout, they are not essential for getting started. Many isometric exercises can be performed effectively using only your body weight and proper technique. As you become more experienced and comfortable with isometric exercises, you can consider incorporating equipment to add variety and challenge to your workouts.

Proper Form and Technique

When it comes to isometric exercises, proper form and technique are essential for maximising effectiveness, preventing injuries, and achieving optimal results. By following correct form and technique, you can target the intended muscles, minimise strain on joints, and ensure a safe and efficient workout. Here are some key guidelines to consider for maintaining proper form and technique during isometric exercises:

1. *Alignment:* Pay attention to your body's alignment throughout each exercise. Maintain a neutral spine, keep your shoulders relaxed, and engage your core muscles for stability. Proper alignment promotes effective muscle engagement and reduces the risk of strain or injury.

2. *Muscle Activation:* Focus on engaging and contracting the specific muscles targeted by the exercise. Visualise the muscle groups you are working and consciously activate them during the hold. This mind-muscle connection enhances the effectiveness of the exercise and ensures that the intended muscles are being engaged.

3. Breathing: Practice controlled breathing during isometric exercises. Inhale deeply before initiating the contraction, and exhale slowly as you exert force and hold the position. Controlled breathing helps stabilise the core, oxygenate the muscles, and maintain focus throughout the exercise.

4. Duration and Intensity: Start with shorter holds and gradually increase the duration as your strength and endurance improve. Aim for holds ranging from 10 to 60 seconds, depending on your fitness level and the specific exercise. Additionally, focus on exerting maximal effort during the hold to maximise muscle activation and challenge.

5. Avoid Straining or Overexertion: While it's important to challenge yourself during isometric exercises, avoid straining or overexerting your muscles. Find the balance between pushing your limits and maintaining control. Listen to your body and stop or modify the exercise if you experience sharp pain or discomfort beyond normal muscle fatigue.

6. Progression: As you become more comfortable with the exercises, gradually progress by increasing the intensity, duration, or adding variations. This progressive overload stimulates muscle growth and strength gains over time. However, progress at a pace that allows your body to adapt and avoid overloading the muscles too quickly.

7. *Focus and Mindfulness:* Maintain focus and mindfulness during each exercise. Concentrate on the muscles being worked, the sensations in your body, and the quality of your movement. Mindful execution helps to ensure proper form, maximise muscle activation, and prevent compensation or reliance on other muscle groups.

Remember, it is recommended to consult with a fitness professional or trainer if you're new to isometric exercises or if you have any specific concerns or limitations. They can provide personalised guidance, corrections, and modifications based on your individual needs and goals. By prioritising proper form and technique, you can optimise the benefits of isometric exercises while minimising the risk of injury.

Chapter 3

Targeted Isometric Exercises for Pain Relief

Upper Body Exercises

Shoulder Stabilisation Exercises

Shoulder stabilisation exercises play a crucial role in improving shoulder strength, mobility, and relieving pain in the upper body. These isometric exercises target the muscles surrounding the shoulder joint, enhancing stability and reducing the risk of injury. Here are some effective shoulder stabilisation exercises:

1. Wall Push-up Hold: Stand facing a wall, approximately arm's length away. Place your palms on the wall at shoulder height and shoulder-width apart. Lean forward slightly, engage your core, and press your palms firmly into the wall. Hold this position for 15-30 seconds while maintaining a straight line from your head to your heels. This exercise strengthens the muscles in your chest, shoulders, and upper back, promoting shoulder stability.

2. *Shoulder External Rotation Hold:* Stand or sit with a resistance band secured at waist height. Hold the band with your affected arm and position your elbow at a 90-degree angle, close to your side. Keep your forearm parallel to the floor. Rotate your forearm away from your body, maintaining the 90-degree angle, until you feel a contraction in your shoulder muscles. Hold this position for 15-30 seconds, focusing on the muscles working around the shoulder joint. This exercise targets the rotator cuff muscles, which are vital for shoulder stability.

3. *Scapular Retraction Hold:* Sit or stand with your arms by your sides and your palms facing forward. Gently squeeze your shoulder blades together while keeping your shoulders relaxed and down. Hold this position for 15-30 seconds, feeling the contraction between your shoulder blades. This exercise strengthens the muscles of the upper back and promotes proper alignment and stability of the shoulders.

4. *Prone Y-T-W Holds:* Lie face down on an exercise mat with your arms extended overhead, forming a Y shape with your thumbs pointing upward. Lift your chest, head, and arms slightly off the ground while maintaining a neutral neck position. Hold this position for 15-30 seconds, focusing on squeezing your shoulder blades together and activating the muscles of the upper back. This exercise targets the muscles responsible for scapular stabilisation and improved posture.

When performing these shoulder stabilisation exercises, remember to maintain proper form and technique. Avoid straining or compensating with other muscle groups. Start with shorter holds and gradually increase the duration as you become more comfortable and stronger. If you experience any pain or discomfort, stop the exercise and consult with a healthcare professional.

Incorporating these targeted shoulder stabilisation exercises into your routine can help alleviate pain, improve shoulder function, and enhance overall upper body strength. Consistency and proper execution are key to reaping the benefits of these isometric exercises.

Chest and Arm Strengthening Exercises

In addition to shoulder stabilisation exercises, incorporating chest and arm strengthening exercises into your isometric workout routine can help relieve pain and improve the strength and function of your upper body. These exercises target the muscles in the chest, arms, and shoulders, promoting stability and reducing discomfort. Here are some effective chest and arm strengthening isometric exercises:

1. *Push-Up Hold:* Assume a push-up position with your hands slightly wider than shoulder-width apart, arms fully extended, and toes on the ground. Lower your body halfway down, keeping your elbows close to your sides. Hold this position for 15-30 seconds, maintaining a straight line from your head to your heels. This exercise engages the muscles in your chest, shoulders, and triceps, promoting upper body strength and stability.

2. *Chest Press Hold:* Sit or stand with a resistance band secured at chest height. Grasp the handles of the band and position your arms in front of you, elbows bent at a 90-degree angle. Push the handles away from your body, straightening your arms while maintaining tension in the band. Hold this position for 15-30 seconds, feeling the contraction in your chest and arms. This exercise targets the muscles of the chest, specifically the pectoralis major and minor.

3. *Bicep Curl Hold:* Stand with your feet shoulder-width apart and hold a dumbbell in each hand, palms facing forward. Keep your elbows close to your sides and curl the dumbbells towards your shoulders. Hold this position for 15-30 seconds, focusing on the contraction in your biceps. This exercise targets the muscles of the upper arms, particularly the biceps brachii.

4. *Tricep Extension Hold:* Stand with your feet shoulder-width apart and hold a dumbbell with both hands overhead. Bend your elbows, lowering the dumbbell behind your head. Hold this position for 15-30 seconds, feeling the contraction in your triceps. This exercise targets the muscles at the back of your upper arms, the triceps brachii.

Remember to maintain proper form and technique during these exercises. Keep your core engaged, avoid straining or using momentum, and breathe steadily throughout the holds. Start with shorter durations and gradually increase as you build strength and confidence. If you experience any pain or discomfort, stop the exercise and consult with a healthcare professional.

Incorporating these targeted chest and arm strengthening isometric exercises into your routine can contribute to pain relief, improve upper body strength, and enhance functional fitness. As with any exercise program, consistency and proper execution are key to achieving desired results.

Core and Back Exercises

In addition to shoulder stabilisation and chest and arm strengthening exercises, incorporating core and back exercises into your isometric workout routine can provide further pain relief and improve the stability and strength of your upper body. These exercises target the muscles in your core and back, promoting better posture and reducing discomfort. Here are some effective core and back isometric exercises:

1. Plank Hold: Start by assuming a push-up position with your forearms on the ground and elbows directly under your shoulders. Engage your core, squeeze your glutes, and maintain a straight line from your head to your heels. Hold this position for 15-30 seconds, focusing on maintaining proper alignment and engaging your abdominal muscles. The plank exercise targets the muscles in your core, including the rectus abdominis, transverse abdominis, and obliques.

2. Superman Hold: Lie face down on an exercise mat with your arms extended overhead and your legs straight. Lift your chest, arms, and legs off the ground simultaneously, engaging your back muscles. Hold this position for 15-30 seconds, feeling the contraction in your lower back and glutes. The superman exercise strengthens the muscles in your lower back and promotes better spinal alignment.

3. *Side Plank Hold:* Lie on your side with your elbow directly under your shoulder and your legs stacked on top of each other. Lift your hips off the ground, creating a straight line from your head to your feet. Hold this position for 15-30 seconds on each side, focusing on engaging your side abdominal muscles and maintaining stability. The side plank exercise targets the obliques and deep core muscles, promoting lateral stability and balance.

4. *Bridge Hold:* Lie on your back with your knees bent and feet flat on the ground, hip-width apart. Press your feet into the ground, engage your glutes, and lift your hips off the ground, creating a straight line from your knees to your shoulders. Hold this position for 15-30 seconds, feeling the contraction in your glutes and lower back. The bridge exercise strengthens the posterior chain muscles, including the glutes and hamstrings, while also engaging the core.

Quadriceps and Hamstring Exercises

Targeting the muscles of the lower body is crucial for achieving overall pain relief and improving strength and stability. Specifically, engaging the quadriceps and hamstrings can help alleviate discomfort and promote balanced muscle development. Here are some effective isometric exercises for the quadriceps and hamstrings:

1. Wall Sit Hold: Stand with your back against a wall and slide down until your knees are bent at a 90-degree angle, as if sitting in an imaginary chair. Ensure your knees are directly above your ankles and your back is pressed against the wall. Hold this position for 15-30 seconds, engaging your quadriceps. The wall sit exercise is an excellent isometric exercise for strengthening the quadriceps, glutes, and lower body muscles.

2. Leg Extension Hold: Sit on a chair or bench with your back supported and your feet flat on the floor. Lift one leg straight in front of you, contracting your quadriceps. Hold this position for 15-30 seconds, focusing on the contraction in your quadriceps. Switch legs and repeat. The leg extension hold targets the quadriceps muscles, promoting strength and stability in the front of the thigh.

3. *Hamstring Curl Hold:* Stand facing a wall or stable surface, holding onto it for support. Bend one knee and lift your foot towards your glutes, contracting your hamstring muscles. Hold this position for 15-30 seconds, feeling the contraction in your hamstrings. Repeat with the other leg. The hamstring curl hold is an effective isometric exercise for strengthening the hamstrings and improving lower body stability.

4. *Single-Leg Glute Bridge Hold:* Lie on your back with your knees bent and feet flat on the ground, hip-width apart. Lift one leg off the ground and extend it straight in front of you. Press through your heel and lift your hips off the ground, engaging your glutes and hamstrings. Hold this position for 15-30 seconds, focusing on the contraction in your glutes and hamstrings. Switch legs and repeat. The single-leg glute bridge hold targets the gluteal muscles and hamstrings while promoting hip stability.

Maintain proper form and technique during these exercises. Ensure your knees are aligned with your ankles and avoid excessive strain or discomfort. Start with shorter durations and gradually increase the hold times as you build strength. If you experience any pain or discomfort, discontinue the exercise and consult with a healthcare professional.

Glutes and Hip Exercises

Engaging the glutes and hip muscles is essential for pain relief and promoting strength and stability in the lower body. By incorporating isometric exercises that target these muscle groups, you can alleviate discomfort and improve overall lower body function. Here are some effective glutes and hip isometric exercises:

1. Glute Bridge Hold: Lie on your back with your knees bent and feet flat on the ground, hip-width apart. Press through your heels and lift your hips off the ground, squeezing your glutes at the top of the movement. Hold this position for 15-30 seconds, focusing on the contraction in your glutes. The glute bridge exercise strengthens the gluteal muscles while also engaging the core and hamstrings.

2. Clamshell Hold: Lie on your side with your knees bent and stacked on top of each other. Keep your feet together and lift your top knee while keeping your feet touching. Hold this position for 15-30 seconds, feeling the contraction in your glutes. Switch sides and repeat. The clamshell exercise targets the gluteus medius, a muscle responsible for hip stability and support.

3. Fire Hydrant Hold: Start on all fours with your hands directly under your shoulders and your knees under your hips. Lift one knee out to the side while keeping it bent at a 90-degree angle. Hold this position for 15-30 seconds, focusing on engaging your glutes. Repeat with the other leg. The fire hydrant exercise targets the glutes and hip muscles, promoting stability and mobility in the hips.

4. Side-Lying Hip Abduction Hold: Lie on your side with your legs extended and stacked on top of each other. Lift your top leg upward, keeping it straight and in line with your body. Hold this position for 15-30 seconds, feeling the contraction in your hip muscles. Switch sides and repeat. The side-lying hip abduction exercise targets the hip abductor muscles, which are essential for hip stability and balance.

Maintain proper form and technique during these exercises. Focus on activating the glutes and hip muscles, and avoid excessive strain or discomfort. Begin with shorter hold times and gradually increase the duration as you build strength. If you experience any pain or discomfort, discontinue the exercise and consult with a healthcare professional.

Calf and Ankle Strengthening Exercises

Strengthening the muscles in your calves and ankles is vital for pain relief and improving lower body stability and mobility. By incorporating isometric exercises that target these muscle groups, you can alleviate discomfort and enhance overall lower body function. Here are some effective calf and ankle strengthening isometric exercises:

1. *Calf Raise Hold:* Stand with your feet hip-width apart near a wall or sturdy support for balance. Rise up onto the balls of your feet, lifting your heels as high as possible. Hold this position for 15-30 seconds, feeling the contraction in your calf muscles. The calf raise exercise strengthens the gastrocnemius and soleus muscles in the calves, promoting ankle stability and strength.

2. *Toe Raise Hold:* Sit on a chair with your feet flat on the ground. Lift your toes up toward your shins, keeping your heels planted on the floor. Hold this position for 15-30 seconds, focusing on the contraction in your shins and ankles. The toe raise exercise targets the muscles in the front of your lower legs, specifically the tibialis anterior, which helps maintain balance and prevent shin splints.

3. Ankle Inversion Hold: Sit on a chair with your feet flat on the ground. Lift the inner edge of your foot, rolling it inward, as if trying to touch the inner arch of your foot to the floor. Hold this position for 15-30 seconds, feeling the contraction along the outer side of your lower leg and ankle. Repeat with the other foot. The ankle inversion exercise targets the muscles responsible for controlling inward ankle movement, promoting ankle stability.

4. Ankle Eversion Hold: Sit on a chair with your feet flat on the ground. Lift the outer edge of your foot, rolling it outward, as if trying to touch the outer edge of your foot to the floor. Hold this position for 15-30 seconds, feeling the contraction along the inner side of your lower leg and ankle. Repeat with the other foot. The ankle eversion exercise targets the muscles responsible for controlling outward ankle movement, enhancing ankle stability.

Planks and Bridging Exercises

Engaging in full-body isometric exercises can provide comprehensive pain relief and promote overall strength and stability throughout your body. Planks and bridging exercises are excellent options to target multiple muscle groups simultaneously. These exercises engage the core, upper body, and lower body muscles, contributing to improved posture, increased strength, and reduced discomfort. Here are some effective full-body isometric exercises:

1. High Plank Hold: Start in a push-up position with your hands directly under your shoulders and your body in a straight line from head to heels. Engage your core, squeeze your glutes, and hold this position for 15-30 seconds, focusing on maintaining proper alignment. The high plank exercise targets the core, shoulders, arms, and leg muscles, providing overall body strength and stability.

2. Low Plank Hold: Begin by resting on your forearms with your elbows directly under your shoulders. Extend your legs back, balancing on your toes. Engage your core, squeeze your glutes, and hold this position for 15-30 seconds, maintaining a straight line from head to heels. The low plank exercise targets the core muscles, including the rectus abdominis, transverse abdominis, and obliques, while also engaging the shoulders and legs.

3. Bridge Hold: Lie on your back with your knees bent and feet flat on the ground, hip-width apart. Press your feet into the ground, engage your glutes, and lift your hips off the ground, creating a straight line from your knees to your shoulders. Hold this position for 15-30 seconds, feeling the contraction in your glutes and lower back. The bridge exercise strengthens the posterior chain muscles, including the glutes, hamstrings, and lower back, while also engaging the core.

4. Side Plank Hold: Lie on your side with your elbow directly under your shoulder and your legs stacked on top of each other. Lift your hips off the ground, creating a straight line from your head to your feet. Hold this position for 15-30 seconds on each side, focusing on engaging your side abdominal muscles and maintaining stability. The side plank exercise targets the obliques, deep core muscles, and shoulders, promoting lateral stability and balance.

Wall Sits and Squats

To engage multiple muscle groups and achieve comprehensive pain relief, incorporating isometric exercises like wall sits and squats into your routine is highly beneficial. These exercises target the lower body, core, and even the upper body, contributing to improved strength, stability, and reduced discomfort. Here are some effective full-body isometric exercises:

1. Wall Sit: Stand with your back against a wall and slide down until your knees are bent at a 90-degree angle, as if sitting in an imaginary chair. Keep your back straight against the wall and hold this position for 15-30 seconds, engaging your quadriceps, hamstrings, and glutes. The wall sit exercise strengthens the lower body muscles, including the quadriceps and glutes, while also engaging the core.

2. Squat Hold: Stand with your feet shoulder-width apart, toes slightly turned out. Lower your hips back and down, as if sitting back into a chair, while keeping your chest up and your knees aligned with your toes. Hold the squat position for 15-30 seconds, engaging your quadriceps, hamstrings, glutes, and core muscles. The squat hold targets the lower body muscles, particularly the quadriceps, hamstrings, and glutes, while also engaging the core and upper body for stability.

3. *Sumo Squat Hold:* Stand with your feet wider than shoulder-width apart, toes pointed slightly outward. Lower your hips down into a deep squat position, keeping your chest up and your knees aligned with your toes. Hold this position for 15-30 seconds, feeling the engagement in your inner thighs, quadriceps, hamstrings, glutes, and core. The sumo squat hold is an effective isometric exercise for targeting the lower body muscles, especially the inner thighs and glutes, while also engaging the core and upper body.

4. *Goblet Squat Hold:* Hold a dumbbell, kettlebell, or any weighted object close to your chest, with your elbows pointing down. Perform a squat by lowering your hips back and down, maintaining an upright posture. Hold the squat position for 15-30 seconds, feeling the engagement in your quadriceps, hamstrings, glutes, core, and upper body. The goblet squat hold not only targets the lower body muscles but also strengthens the upper body and core due to the added weight.

Push-ups and Variations

Push-ups are excellent full-body isometric exercises that engage multiple muscle groups, including the chest, shoulders, arms, core, and even the lower body. Incorporating different variations of push-ups into your routine can provide comprehensive pain relief, improve upper body strength, and enhance overall body stability. Here are some effective push-up variations:

1. Standard Push-up: Start in a high plank position with your hands slightly wider than shoulder-width apart and your body in a straight line from head to heels. Lower your chest toward the ground while keeping your elbows close to your sides. Push back up to the starting position. Perform 8-12 repetitions or hold the lowered position for 15-30 seconds to engage the muscles isometrically.

2. Incline Push-up: Place your hands on an elevated surface, such as a bench or step, while maintaining a straight line from head to heels. Perform the push-up movement, lowering your chest toward the elevated surface and then pushing back up. The incline push-up is a modified version that reduces the amount of body weight being lifted, making it slightly easier than the standard push-up.

3. Decline Push-up: Place your feet on an elevated surface, such as a step or sturdy platform, with your hands on the ground in a high plank position. Perform the push-up movement, lowering your chest toward the ground and then pushing back up. The decline push-up increases the challenge by elevating your feet, engaging the chest, shoulders, and triceps to a greater extent.

4. Diamond Push-up: Assume a standard push-up position, but place your hands close together, forming a diamond shape with your thumbs and index fingers. Perform the push-up movement, lowering your chest toward the diamond shape and pushing back up. The diamond push-up targets the triceps and inner chest muscles, providing a unique challenge to the upper body.

5. One-Legged Push-up: Start in a standard push-up position and lift one leg off the ground, extending it straight behind you. Perform the push-up movement, lowering your chest toward the ground and pushing back up while keeping one leg elevated. Switch legs and repeat. The one-legged push-up adds an additional challenge by engaging the core and lower body for stability.

Chapter 4

Designing an Isometric Exercise Program

Setting Goals and Tracking Progress

When embarking on an isometric exercise program for pain relief and overall strength, it is essential to set clear goals and track your progress. Setting goals provides direction and motivation, while tracking progress allows you to monitor your advancements and make necessary adjustments. Here are some steps to help you establish goals and track your progress effectively:

1. Define Your Objectives: Determine what you want to achieve through your isometric exercise program. Are you aiming to alleviate specific pain or discomfort? Do you want to improve overall strength, endurance, or mobility? Establish clear and realistic goals that are specific, measurable, attainable, relevant, and time-bound (SMART goals).

2. *Assess Your Current Fitness Level:* Conduct a self-assessment of your current fitness level to gauge your starting point. Consider factors such as strength, flexibility, and overall physical condition. This assessment will help you set realistic goals and tailor your program to your individual needs.

3. *Plan Your Exercise Program:* Based on your goals and fitness assessment, design an isometric exercise program that includes a variety of exercises targeting different muscle groups. Determine the frequency, duration, and intensity of your workouts. Gradually progress the difficulty level and increase the duration of your holds over time to challenge your muscles and promote continuous improvement.

4. *Track Your Progress:* Keep a record of your workouts, including the exercises performed, hold times, and any variations or modifications. Additionally, track how you feel before and after each session, noting any changes in pain or discomfort levels. Regularly reassess your fitness level to evaluate your progress and adjust your program accordingly.

5. *Monitor Performance Indicators:* Alongside tracking your exercises, monitor performance indicators such as increased hold times, improved form and technique, increased muscle strength, and reduced pain or discomfort levels. These indicators will help you gauge your progress and provide motivation as you witness tangible improvements.

6. *Adapt and Adjust:* As you progress in your isometric exercise program, periodically reassess your goals and make necessary adjustments to keep challenging yourself. Modify exercises, increase hold times, or introduce new variations to prevent plateaus and continue making strides toward your objectives.

7. *Seek Professional Guidance:* If needed, consult with a fitness professional, physical therapist, or healthcare provider who can provide guidance and ensure your exercise program aligns with your specific needs and limitations.

Creating a Balanced Routine

When designing an isometric exercise program, it is crucial to create a balanced routine that targets different muscle groups and promotes overall strength, endurance, and pain relief. A well-rounded program ensures that all areas of your body are adequately engaged and avoids overemphasis on certain muscles. Here are some key considerations for creating a balanced isometric exercise routine:

1. Upper Body Exercises: Include a variety of isometric exercises that target the muscles in your upper body, such as the chest, shoulders, arms, and back. This can involve exercises like planks, push-ups, wall sits, and variations of these movements. Distribute the workload evenly across different muscle groups to achieve a balanced routine.

2. Lower Body Exercises: Incorporate isometric exercises that focus on the lower body, including the quadriceps, hamstrings, glutes, and calves. Exercises like squats, lunges, wall sits, and leg lifts can effectively engage these muscle groups. Aim for a balance between exercises that target the front and back of the legs to maintain muscular equilibrium.

3. *Core and Abdominal Exercises:* Strengthening the core is crucial for stability and overall body strength. Include isometric exercises like planks, side planks, and bridges to engage the abdominal muscles, obliques, and lower back. These exercises contribute to better posture, spinal support, and pain relief in the core region.

4. *Balance and Stability Exercises:* Add exercises that enhance balance and stability, such as single-leg stands, single-leg squats, and bird-dog exercises. These movements target smaller stabilising muscles and help prevent imbalances or injuries caused by muscular asymmetries.

5. *Full Body Exercises:* Incorporate full-body isometric exercises like high-intensity interval training (HIIT) or circuit training that engage multiple muscle groups simultaneously. These exercises can involve a combination of movements like burpees, mountain climbers, or kettlebell swings, challenging your entire body and promoting overall fitness.

6. *Rest and Recovery:* Allow for adequate rest and recovery between workout sessions. Isometric exercises can be demanding on the muscles, so it's essential to give your body time to repair and rebuild. Consider incorporating rest days into your routine or alternating between upper body and lower body workouts to prevent overexertion.

7. *Progression and Variation:* As you become stronger and more comfortable with your routine, progressively increase the difficulty level of your exercises. This can be achieved by extending hold times, adding resistance, or trying advanced variations of the exercises. Introduce new exercises periodically to keep your routine fresh and challenging.

8. *Listen to Your Body:* Pay attention to your body's signals and modify exercises or hold times if you experience discomfort or pain. Everyone's fitness level and capabilities are unique, so it's crucial to tailor the routine to your individual needs and limitations.

By creating a balanced isometric exercise routine that targets all major muscle groups and incorporates variety, you can maximise the benefits of your program and achieve optimal pain relief, strength, and endurance. Remember to consult with a healthcare professional or fitness expert if you have any specific concerns or medical conditions that may require additional guidance.

Incorporating Isometric Exercises into Your Daily Life

To maximise the benefits of isometric exercises and promote pain relief, strength, and endurance, it is essential to incorporate them into your daily life beyond structured workout sessions. By integrating isometric exercises into your routine, you can enhance muscular engagement, maintain flexibility, and improve overall well-being. Here are some tips for incorporating isometric exercises into your daily life:

1. Seize Everyday Opportunities: Look for opportunities throughout the day to engage your muscles isometrically. For example, while standing in line or waiting for an appointment, perform calf raises by lifting your heels off the ground and holding the position for a few seconds. Engage your core muscles by practicing abdominal contractions while sitting at your desk or watching TV.

2. Active Sitting: If you have a sedentary job or spend long hours sitting, make it a habit to incorporate isometric exercises into your sitting routine. Perform seated leg extensions by lifting one leg off the ground and holding it straight out in front of you for a few seconds. Engage your core by sitting tall and tightening your abdominal muscles while maintaining good posture.

3. *Household Chores:* Turn everyday household chores into opportunities for isometric exercises. Engage your muscles by maintaining a tight grip and contracting your arm muscles while carrying groceries or lifting objects. When vacuuming, focus on engaging your core and maintaining an upright posture. Squat or lunge while doing activities like gardening or cleaning low surfaces to engage your lower body muscles.

4. *Commute Smartly:* If you commute to work or travel frequently, use your travel time creatively. While sitting on a bus or train, perform seated isometric exercises like glute squeezes or thigh contractions. If you drive, engage your core muscles by practising abdominal contractions and sitting tall.

5. *Stair Workouts:* Take advantage of stairs in your daily routine. Instead of taking the elevator or escalator, opt for the stairs whenever possible. Incorporate stair exercises such as calf raises, step-ups, or using the stairs for balance while performing lunges or squats.

6. *Stretch and Hold:* Incorporate isometric stretches into your daily stretching routine. After a warm-up, stretch a muscle group and hold the stretch for an extended duration, usually around 30 seconds. Isometric stretching can improve flexibility and range of motion while engaging the targeted muscles.

7. *Break-Time Exercise:* Take short breaks throughout the day to perform isometric exercises. Set a reminder to stand up and do wall sits, push-ups against a wall, or plank holds. These quick bursts of activity can energize your body, improve circulation, and alleviate stiffness.

8. *Mindful Movement:* Practise mindfulness during daily activities. Whether you're brushing your teeth, washing dishes, or waiting for the microwave, use these moments to focus on your posture and engage your muscles. Stand tall, contract your abdominal muscles, and maintain good alignment.

By incorporating isometric exercises into your daily life, you can make significant progress toward your goals and improve overall strength and endurance. Remember to start gradually, listen to your body, and adjust the exercises to your fitness level. With consistency and creativity, you can turn ordinary moments into opportunities for building strength and promoting pain relief.

Progressive Overload and Intensity

Once you have established a foundation with isometric exercises and built strength and endurance, it's time to explore advanced techniques and variations to continue challenging your muscles and making progress. Progressive overload and intensity are key principles to incorporate into your isometric exercise routine to stimulate further growth and maximise results. Here are some strategies for implementing progressive overload and increasing the intensity of your workouts:

1. Increase Hold Times: Gradually increase the duration of your isometric holds. Begin by adding a few seconds to your current hold times, and as your muscles adapt, continue progressing incrementally. This progressive increase in hold times challenges your muscles and promotes strength gains over time.

2. Add Resistance: Introduce external resistance to your isometric exercises to intensify the workload on your muscles. You can use resistance bands, weights, or even your body weight by positioning yourself at an angle that creates additional resistance. For example, during a wall sit, you can hold a medicine ball or place a weight plate on your thighs.

3. *Incorporate Isometric Contractions:* Instead of holding a static position, include dynamic isometric contractions within your exercises. For instance, during a plank, perform small movements such as shoulder taps, leg lifts, or knee drives while maintaining a stable core and engaged muscles. These contractions enhance muscle activation and challenge your stability.

4. *Eccentric Isometrics:* Explore eccentric isometric exercises, which involve controlled lengthening of the muscle while maintaining an isometric contraction. For example, during a push-up, lower yourself slowly to the ground while maintaining tension in your muscles, and then push back up. This combination of eccentric and isometric contractions can promote muscle growth and increase strength.

5. *Unilateral Exercises:* Focus on unilateral exercises to address muscle imbalances and further challenge your stabilising muscles. Perform isometric exercises using one limb at a time, such as single-leg wall sits, one-arm planks, or single-leg calf raises. Unilateral exercises not only improve overall strength but also enhance balance and stability.

6. ***Plyometric Isometrics:*** Integrate plyometric movements into your isometric exercises to incorporate power and explosiveness. For instance, perform a jump squat and hold the squat position isometrically for a few seconds before repeating the jump. Plyometric isometrics can enhance muscular power, coordination, and dynamic strength.

7. ***Variations and Progressions:*** Continuously introduce new variations and progressions to your existing exercises. For example, modify the hand position during a push-up by placing them wider or closer together. Increase the difficulty of a wall sit by elevating one foot or performing the exercise on an unstable surface like a balance board. These variations keep your workouts challenging and prevent plateauing.

Remember to listen to your body and progress gradually to avoid overexertion or injury. Incorporating progressive overload and increasing intensity should be a gradual process that allows your muscles to adapt and grow stronger over time. Keep track of your progress, adjust your workouts accordingly, and seek guidance from a fitness professional if needed.

Isometric Exercises with Resistance Bands

Incorporating resistance bands into your isometric exercise routine is an excellent way to add variety, challenge your muscles, and enhance the effectiveness of your workouts. Resistance bands provide adjustable resistance throughout the range of motion, making them a versatile tool for isometric exercises. Here are some isometric exercises with resistance bands to take your training to the next level:

1. Band Squats: Secure the resistance band under your feet and hold the handles at shoulder height. Assume a squat position with your feet hip-width apart and knees slightly bent. Engage your core, maintain an upright posture, and push against the resistance of the band as you hold the squat position isometrically. This exercise targets your quadriceps, hamstrings, and glutes.

2. Band Rows: Anchor the resistance band to a sturdy object at waist height. Hold the handles with an overhand grip and step back to create tension in the band. Keeping your back straight, engage your core and pull the band toward your body, squeezing your shoulder blades together. Hold the position briefly, focusing on maintaining tension in your back muscles. Band rows primarily target your upper back and biceps.

3. Band Chest Press: Secure the resistance band behind you at chest level. Hold the handles with an overhand grip and step forward to create tension in the band. Stand with feet shoulder-width apart, engage your core, and push the handles forward, extending your arms while keeping your elbows slightly bent. Hold the extended position, feeling the tension in your chest muscles. Band chest presses effectively target your chest and triceps.

4. Band Plank Hold: Place the resistance band around your upper back, just below your shoulder blades. Assume a plank position with your forearms on the ground and elbows directly beneath your shoulders. Engage your core, squeeze your glutes, and press against the resistance of the band, maintaining a straight line from your head to your heels. This exercise intensifies the activation of your core muscles.

5. Band Lateral Leg Lift: Secure the resistance band around your ankles or just above your knees. Stand with feet hip-width apart, engage your core, and lift one leg out to the side while keeping the other leg stable. Hold the lifted leg at the highest point and resist against the band's tension. This exercise targets your hip abductors and helps strengthen your glutes and outer thighs.

6. *Band Shoulder Press:* Step on the resistance band and hold the handles at shoulder height. Stand with feet shoulder-width apart, engage your core, and push the handles upward, extending your arms while keeping your elbows slightly bent. Hold the extended position and resist against the resistance of the band. Band shoulder presses focus on your deltoids, triceps, and upper back muscles.

7. *Band Calf Raises:* Place the resistance band under the balls of your feet and hold the handles at your sides. Stand with feet hip-width apart, engage your core, and rise up onto your tiptoes, lifting your heels as high as possible. Hold the lifted position, feeling the resistance from the band, and squeeze your calf muscles. Band calf raises target your calves and help improve lower leg strength.

When performing isometric exercises with resistance bands, maintain proper form, control the movements, and focus on contracting the targeted muscles throughout each hold. Gradually increase the resistance of the band as your muscles adapt and grow stronger.

Combining Isometric Exercises with Stretching and Mobility Work

To enhance the effectiveness of your isometric exercise routine and promote overall flexibility and mobility, it is beneficial to incorporate stretching and mobility exercises. Stretching helps lengthen the muscles and improve their range of motion, while mobility exercises focus on joint mobility and movement patterns. By combining these practices with isometric exercises, you can optimise your training and experience a well-rounded fitness regimen. Here's how you can combine isometric exercises with stretching and mobility work:

1. Pre-Isometric Warm-up: Before engaging in isometric exercises, perform a dynamic warm-up routine that includes mobility exercises and active stretches. This prepares your muscles and joints for the upcoming isometric holds and reduces the risk of injury. Incorporate exercises such as leg swings, arm circles, hip rotations, and shoulder rotations to warm up the major muscle groups and increase blood flow.

2. *Isometric Stretch Holds:* After completing a set of isometric exercises, incorporate static stretches to target the specific muscle groups you worked. Hold each stretch for 20-30 seconds, focusing on maintaining proper form and feeling a gentle stretch in the targeted muscles. Examples of isometric stretches include a standing quad stretch, hamstring stretch, chest stretch, and calf stretch. Isometric stretching can improve flexibility and promote muscle relaxation.

3. *Active Mobility Exercises:* Integrate active mobility exercises between sets of isometric exercises to improve joint range of motion and enhance overall mobility. These exercises involve controlled movements that actively engage the muscles and joints. Examples include shoulder circles, hip rotations, ankle circles, and spinal twists. Active mobility exercises help lubricate the joints, improve movement patterns, and prevent stiffness.

4. *Dynamic Stretching Complexes:* Incorporate dynamic stretching complexes that involve flowing movements and continuous muscle activation. These complexes combine multiple stretches and movements into a fluid sequence. For instance, perform a series of lunges with overhead reaches, incorporating side bends and rotations. Dynamic stretching complexes increase flexibility, improve coordination, and warm up the muscles simultaneously.

5. *Post-Workout Stretching:* After completing your isometric exercise routine, allocate time for a comprehensive cool-down that includes static stretching for all major muscle groups. Focus on holding each stretch for 30-60 seconds to promote muscle recovery, decrease muscle soreness, and increase overall flexibility. Include stretches for the chest, shoulders, back, hips, hamstrings, quadriceps, calves, and any other targeted muscle groups.

By combining isometric exercises with stretching and mobility work, you enhance your body's overall functionality, reduce the risk of injury, and promote balanced muscular development. Remember to perform all exercises with proper form and within your comfort level. Adjust the intensity and duration of stretches and mobility exercises based on your individual needs and limitations.

Chapter 6

Tips for Maximising Results and Avoiding Common Mistakes

Breathing Techniques and Mental Focus

While performing isometric exercises, proper breathing techniques and mental focus play a crucial role in maximising your results and ensuring safety and effectiveness. By incorporating specific breathing patterns and maintaining mental focus, you can optimise your performance and reap the benefits of your isometric exercise routine. Here are some tips to help you master breathing techniques and develop mental focus:

1. Diaphragmatic Breathing: Practise diaphragmatic breathing, also known as belly breathing or deep breathing. Instead of shallow chest breathing, focus on inhaling deeply through your nose, allowing your abdomen to expand fully, and exhaling slowly through your mouth. This type of breathing promotes relaxation, oxygenates your muscles, and enhances overall stability during isometric holds.

2. *Coordination of Breathing and Contraction:* Coordinate your breathing with the contraction and release of muscles during isometric exercises. Generally, exhale during the exertion phase or when contracting the targeted muscles and inhale during the relaxation phase or when releasing the tension. This coordinated breathing pattern helps maintain stability, control, and efficient muscle activation.

3. *Maintain Mental Focus:* Concentrate on the muscles you are targeting during each isometric exercise. Visualise the muscles contracting and engaging, fostering a mind-muscle connection. By directing your attention to the specific muscles you are working, you enhance muscle recruitment and overall effectiveness of the exercise. Mental focus also aids in maintaining proper form and technique.

4. *Mindful Awareness of Tension:* Develop mindful awareness of muscle tension throughout your body during isometric exercises. Pay attention to any areas of excessive tension or unnecessary muscle engagement. Relax those muscles and redirect the tension to the targeted muscles. Mindful awareness helps optimize muscle activation, prevent compensation, and reduce the risk of strain or injury.

5. *Mental Imagery and Visualization:* Utilise mental imagery and visualisation techniques to enhance your performance and motivation during isometric exercises. Create a mental image of successfully completing the exercise with perfect form, feeling the muscles working and getting stronger. Visualise yourself achieving your fitness goals and imagine the positive impact of your efforts on your overall well-being.

6. *Incorporate Mindfulness or Meditation Practices:* Consider integrating mindfulness or meditation practices into your isometric exercise routine. Prioritise present-moment awareness, non-judgmental observation of sensations, and a calm and focused mindset. This can help reduce stress, improve concentration, and enhance your overall training experience.

Common Pitfalls and How to Overcome Them

While engaging in isometric exercises, it's important to be aware of common pitfalls that may hinder your progress or increase the risk of injury. By understanding these pitfalls and implementing strategies to overcome them, you can optimise your training experience and achieve better results. Here are some common pitfalls and tips on how to overcome them:

1. Holding Your Breath: One common mistake during isometric exercises is holding your breath or breathing irregularly. This can lead to increased muscle tension and decreased oxygen supply to your muscles. To overcome this, focus on maintaining a steady breathing pattern throughout each exercise. Breathe deeply and rhythmically, coordinating your breath with muscle contractions and releases.

2. Poor Posture and Alignment: Incorrect posture and alignment can reduce the effectiveness of isometric exercises and increase the risk of strain or injury. Ensure that you maintain proper form and alignment for each exercise. Pay attention to your posture, keeping your spine straight, shoulders relaxed, and core engaged. Seek guidance from a fitness professional or use mirrors to check your form.

3. Overexertion and Overtraining: Pushing yourself too hard or overtraining can lead to muscle fatigue, diminished performance, and potential injuries. It's essential to listen to your body and respect its limits. Gradually progress in intensity and duration, allowing sufficient rest and recovery between workouts. Incorporate rest days and consider incorporating active recovery exercises to promote muscle repair and prevent overexertion.

4. Neglecting Proper Warm-up and Cool-down: Skipping warm-up exercises and cool-down stretches can increase the risk of injury and hinder your performance. Prioritize a dynamic warm-up routine before your isometric exercises to prepare your muscles and joints. Likewise, include a comprehensive cool-down that incorporates static stretching to promote muscle recovery and flexibility.

5. Lack of Variety and Progression: Repeating the same isometric exercises without adding variety or increasing the challenge can lead to plateaus and diminished results. Incorporate different exercises that target various muscle groups and consider using props or resistance bands to add variety and progression. Gradually increase the intensity, duration, or difficulty of your exercises to continually challenge your muscles.

6. Insufficient Rest and Recovery: Rest and recovery are vital components of any training program. Adequate rest allows your muscles to repair and grow stronger. Avoid the pitfall of overtraining by incorporating rest days into your routine. Additionally, prioritize quality sleep, proper nutrition, and hydration to support your body's recovery process.

7. Lack of Patience and Consistency: Achieving significant results with isometric exercises takes time and consistency. It's essential to set realistic goals and understand that progress may be gradual. Stay committed to your routine and maintain consistency in your workouts. Celebrate small milestones along the way to stay motivated and encouraged.

Listening to Your Body and Adapting the Exercises

One of the most important aspects of any fitness routine, including isometric exercises, is listening to your body and adapting the exercises according to your individual needs.

1. Recognize Sensations: During isometric exercises, be mindful of the sensations in your body. Pay attention to feelings of discomfort, pain, or excessive strain. It's normal to feel some muscle fatigue and challenge during the exercises, but it's important to distinguish between normal sensations and potential signs of injury or overexertion.

2. Modify Intensity: If you experience discomfort or pain during an exercise, it's essential to modify the intensity to a level that is more comfortable for you. Reduce the duration or intensity of the hold, or adjust the range of motion to a position that doesn't cause pain. You can gradually progress the intensity as your body becomes stronger and more accustomed to the exercises.

3. Respect Limitations: Understand and respect your body's limitations. If you have a pre-existing injury, chronic condition, or specific physical limitations, consult with a healthcare professional or a qualified fitness trainer who can provide guidance on modifying the exercises to suit your needs. Avoid pushing yourself beyond your comfort level and work within your own capabilities.

4. *Adjust Range of Motion:* Each person has a different range of motion, and it's important to work within your own limits. If you find it challenging to perform certain exercises with a full range of motion, reduce the range or modify the position to a comfortable and safe level. Gradually work on increasing your range of motion over time.

5. *Take Breaks and Rest:* If you feel overly fatigued or exhausted during a workout, it's okay to take breaks and rest as needed. Don't push through extreme discomfort or fatigue. Allow your body time to recover between sets or exercises, and listen to your body's signals when it's time to take a break or conclude your workout.

6. *Seek Professional Guidance:* If you're new to isometric exercises or have specific concerns, it's beneficial to seek guidance from a qualified fitness professional. They can provide personalised advice, help you with proper form and technique, and guide you in adapting the exercises to your unique circumstances.

Conclusion

Recap of Key Points

In this book, we have explored the world of isometric exercises for pain relief, focusing on how to build strength and endurance without moving. Let's recap the key points we have covered:

- Isometric exercises involve static muscle contractions without joint movement, making them ideal for pain relief and rehabilitation.
- These exercises provide various benefits, including increased muscle strength, improved joint stability, enhanced posture, and reduced risk of injury.
- Isometric exercises can be performed by anyone, regardless of fitness level or age.
- We have explored a range of targeted isometric exercises for different areas of the body, including the upper body, core and back, and lower body.
- We have also discussed full body isometric exercises that engage multiple muscle groups simultaneously.
- Designing an isometric exercise program involves setting goals, tracking progress, creating a balanced routine, and incorporating exercises into your daily life.

- We have explored advanced techniques such as progressive overload, using resistance bands, and combining isometric exercises with stretching and mobility work.
- Breathing techniques, mental focus, and proper form are essential for maximising results and avoiding common mistakes.
- Lastly, we have emphasised the importance of listening to your body, adapting exercises to your needs, and seeking professional guidance when necessary.

Maintaining a Long-Term Isometric Exercise Practice

To maintain a long-term isometric exercise practice, consistency is key. Make it a habit to incorporate these exercises into your regular routine. Gradually increase the intensity and duration of your workouts as your strength and endurance improve. Remember to listen to your body and adapt the exercises as needed to avoid injury and achieve optimal results. Stay motivated by setting realistic goals, celebrating your progress, and seeking support from a fitness community or professional.

Final Thoughts and Encouragement

Incorporating isometric exercises into your life can have a transformative impact on your well-being. These exercises offer a unique approach to pain relief, strength building, and endurance training. By consistently practising isometric exercises, you can improve your physical fitness, enhance your body's resilience, and experience greater overall health and vitality.

As you embark on your isometric exercise journey, remember to be patient with yourself and enjoy the process. Each small step you take towards your goals is significant. Stay committed, stay focused, and always listen to your body. With dedication and perseverance, you have the power to unlock your potential and lead a life free from pain and discomfort.

Best wishes on your isometric exercise adventure. May it bring you strength, relief, and a renewed sense of well-being.